ASHITABA FOR BEGINNERS

Unlocking The Healing Power Of Ashitaba, A Comprehensive Guide To Boosting Your Health, Enhancing Vitality, And Embracing Nature's Wellness And Longevity

Georgette Lockett

DISCLAIMER

The author of this book is not affiliated, associated, endorsed, sponsored, or approved by any company or individual. The views and opinions expressed in this book are solely those of the author and do not necessarily reflect the official policy or position of any entity.

The author hereby disclaims any relationship, collaboration, or partnership with any company or individual mentioned in this book. Any references to products, services, or individuals are provided for informational purposes only and should not be construed as an endorsement or recommendation.

Readers are advised to exercise their own judgment and discretion when applying the information provided in this book. The author shall not be held responsible for any actions taken by readers based on the content of this book.

This book is intended for general informational purposes only, and the author makes no representations or warranties of any kind, express or implied, about the completeness, accuracy, reliability, suitability, or availability of the information contained herein. Any reliance on the information in this book is at the reader's own risk.

The author reserves the right to update, change, or modify any information in this book without notice. It is the responsibility of the reader to verify any information before taking any actions based on the content of this book.

By reading this book, the reader acknowledges and agrees to the terms of this disclaimer.

Table of Contents

INTRODUCTION

"Ashitaba: Unveiling Nature's Miracle" delves into the numerous features of the botanical miracle known as Ashitaba to provide a full knowledge of this cherished plant.

Ashitaba, technically known as Angelica keiskei, is a perennial plant native to the Japanese island of Hachijo. This plant is revered in traditional Asian medicine for its brilliant green leaves and rich mythology, as well as its numerous therapeutic effects.

Historical Significance

Ashitaba's historical importance spans generations of Japanese culture and tradition, with origins dating back millennia. It's known as the "Tomorrow's Leaf" because of its quick regeneration after harvesting, and it's linked to stories of longevity and healing in Japanese mythology.

Its longstanding usage in numerous tonics, teas, and health cures emphasizes its historical significance.

Purpose Of The Guide

The goal of this thorough reference is to solve the mystery surrounding Ashitaba by providing an in-depth examination of its botanical, medicinal, and cultural importance. It aims to give an in-depth explanation of the features of Ashitaba, as well as its historical background, present uses, and prospective future developments. This book aims to be an essential resource for students, practitioners, and enthusiasts interested in discovering the mysteries of this extraordinary plant, whether it is researching its historic usage or its rising role in contemporary health.

CHAPTER 1

Botanical Profile

Taxonomy And Classification

Ashitaba, also known technically as Angelica keiskei Koidzumi is a member of the Apiaceae family. This group of fragrant plants has hollow stems and umbelliferous inflorescences. Ashitaba, a perennial herbaceous plant of the Angelica genus, is well-known for its many therapeutic benefits.

Geographic Distribution

Ashitaba is native to Japan's islands, notably the Izu and Hachijojima Islands, although it has been extensively planted in other Asian nations owing to its therapeutic value. Its tolerance to many environmental conditions has led to its expansion outside of Japan.

Morphological Features

Ashitaba is distinguished by its distinctive look, with broad, lobed leaves resembling those of the common maple tree. The plant may reach many feet in height, with a strong stem and vivid green leaves. Its stem and leaf undersides generate a yellow sap rich in phytonutrients, giving it a distinct character. The blooming structure is made up of tiny, clustered yellow-green flowers that generate seeds and allow for spontaneous proliferation.

This chapter covers the classification of Ashitaba, its native environment, and the visual and structural characteristics that distinguish this important plant. Understanding these botanical features gives the groundwork for understanding the many uses and applications mentioned in later chapters.

CHAPTER 2

Nutritional Composition

Ashitaba, technically known as Angelica keiskei Koidzumi, is a Japanese herbaceous plant. Ashitaba has gained popularity in recent years owing to its possible health advantages, in addition to its longstanding usage in folk medicine. In this chapter, we will look at Ashitaba's nutritional content, concentrating on vitamins and minerals, phytonutrients, and antioxidant capabilities.

Vitamins And Minerals

Vitamins:

1. Ashitaba is high in vitamin C (ascorbic acid), an important component renowned for its antioxidant effects. Vitamin C is essential for collagen formation, immunological function, and skin health.

2. Vitamin A (Beta-carotene): Ashitaba contains beta-carotene, a precursor of vitamin A. Vitamin A

is essential for healthy eyesight, immunological function, and skin.

3. Ashitaba includes B vitamins such as B1 (thiamine), B2 (riboflavin), B3 (niacin), B5 (pantothenic acid), and B9 (folate). These vitamins aid in the metabolism of energy, the creation of neurotransmitters, and the repair of DNA.

Minerals:

1. **Potassium:** Potassium is a mineral that is necessary for electrolyte balance, heart health, and blood pressure regulation. Ashitaba includes a high concentration of potassium.

2. **Calcium:** Ashitaba is high in calcium, which is essential for bone health, muscular function, and blood coagulation.

3. **Iron:** Iron is required for hemoglobin production and oxygen transport in the blood. Ashitaba is a good source of dietary iron.

Phytonutrients

Chalcones:

The flavonoids known as chalcones are specific to Ashitaba. Chalcones are anti-inflammatory and antioxidant in nature. These chemicals have been researched for their ability to improve cardiovascular health and lower the risk of chronic illnesses.

Coumarins:

Coumarins, another kind of phytonutrient found in Ashitaba, have been linked to anti-tumor and anti-inflammatory properties. Coumarins, according to research, may add to the herb's potential as a natural medicinal agent.

Polysaccharides:

Polysaccharides in Ashitaba have immunomodulatory effects. These substances may help to improve the body's immunological response and general immune system health.

Antioxidant Properties

Ashitaba has high antioxidant activity because of its high concentration of vitamins (particularly vitamin C and beta-carotene) and phytonutrients. Antioxidants help the body neutralize free radicals, lowering oxidative stress and inflammation. This antioxidative activity adds to Ashitaba's ability to promote general health and avoid chronic illnesses.

Finally, the nutritional makeup of Ashitaba includes a wide range of vitamins, minerals, and phytonutrients, all of which contribute to its potential health benefits. Ashitaba is a great addition to a balanced diet because of its mix of these components, which may boost immunological function, cardiovascular health, and general well-being.

CHAPTER 3

Medicinal Uses

Ashitaba, formally known as Angelica keiskei, is a rare plant with several therapeutic characteristics that have been used in traditional Japanese medicine for centuries. It has garnered great interest for its possible health advantages throughout the years, prompting intensive contemporary research and investigations into its different uses.

Traditional Healing Practices

1. **Japanese Folklore and Traditional Medicine:** Ashitaba has a long cultural history in Japan, where it is treasured as a "longevity herb" for its health-promoting properties. It was largely utilized as a cure for many maladies in traditional Japanese medicine, such as digestive disorders, and skin conditions, and promoting vigor.

2.   Wellness Tonic: It is thought that consuming ashitaba tea or its leaves may cleanse the blood, assist digestion, and boost overall vitality. It was often used as a tonic to improve lifespan and overall well-being.

3.   **Wound Healing and Skin Health:** Because of its reputed antibacterial and wound-healing characteristics, topical treatments of ashitaba were often used to treat wounds, cuts, and skin infections.

Modern Medicinal Applications

1.   **Antioxidant and Anti-inflammatory Properties:** Studies have shown that ashitaba has powerful antioxidant and anti-inflammatory properties due to its high concentration of chalcones, flavonoids, and other bioactive components. These characteristics contribute to its ability to reduce oxidative stress and inflammation in the body.

2. **Immune System Support:** Some research suggests that ashitaba has immunomodulatory properties, which may help the immune system function by increasing the body's natural defensive systems.

3. **Cardioprotective Effects:** A new study suggests that ashitaba may have cardiovascular advantages, including possible support for healthy cholesterol levels and blood pressure via bioactive substances such as chalcones and vitamins.

4. **Anticancer Potential:** Preliminary research has looked at ashitaba's anticancer characteristics, namely its capacity to stop the development of certain cancer cells. However, a more detailed study in this area is required.

Research And Studies

1. **Bioactive chemicals:** Ashitaba contains a variety of bioactive chemicals, including xanthoangelol,

chitin, and coumarins, which contribute to its therapeutic benefits.

2. **Clinical studies:** Ongoing clinical studies seek to further investigate Ashitaba's therapeutic potential in a variety of health diseases, including diabetes, inflammatory disorders, and cancer.

3. **Safety and dose:** Efforts are being conducted to discover the appropriate dose and safety profile of ashitaba, guaranteeing its effectiveness while minimizing side effects.

Finally, the therapeutic benefits of ashitaba range from its historical importance in traditional healing methods to present scientific research. Its wide range of possible health advantages, including antioxidant, anti-inflammatory, and immune-modulating capabilities, has piqued the curiosity of natural medicine and health researchers.

CHAPTER 4

Culinary Uses

Culinary Tradition

In Japanese food and traditional medicine, ashitaba, also known as "Tomorrow's Leaf," is adored. It has been included in a variety of culinary traditions due to its unusual taste character and outstanding nutritional value. This perennial plant is valued not just for its medicinal benefits, but also for its culinary flexibility.

Recipes And Culinary Tips

1. Tempura Ashitaba:

• Composition:

• Ashitaba leaf

• Batter for tempura

• Cooking oil

• Get Ready:

• Tempura batter the ashitaba leaves.

• Fry till golden brown and crispy.

• Accompany with tempura dipping sauce.

2. Salad with ashitaba:

• Composition:

• Ashitaba stems and leaves

• Fresh veggies (cucumbers, tomatoes, and so on).

• Balsamic vinegar with olive oil

• Season with salt and pepper to taste

• Get Ready:

• Chop the ashitaba leaves and stems with the other veggies.

• Toss with olive oil, balsamic vinegar, salt, and pepper.

• Serve as a light salad.

3. Tea Ashitaba:

• Composition:

• Ashitaba leaves, dried

• Warm water

• Get Ready:

• Soak dried ashitaba leaves for a few minutes in boiling water.

• Strain the tea and enjoy the somewhat bitter but refreshing flavor.

Incorporating Ashitaba Into Daily Diet

1. **Smoothies:** For a healthy smoothie, combine fresh ashitaba leaves with fruits such as bananas, cherries, or mangoes.

2. **Soups and broths:** For an extra nutritious boost, add chopped ashitaba leaves to soups or broths.

3. **Stir-Fries:** Combine chopped ashitaba leaves with other vegetables or protein sources in stir-fried recipes.

4. **Baked Goods:** For a distinctive taste twist, try incorporating dried and powdered ashitaba leaves into muffin or pancake batter.

Culinary Advantages

• **Nutritious Powerhouse:** Ashitaba is high in vitamins (A, B, C, E) and minerals (potassium, calcium, iron), giving recipes a significant nutritious boost.

• **Distinctive Flavor:** It has a somewhat bitter taste with herbaceous undertones, giving it a distinct flavor to a variety of culinary creations.

• **Versatile Ingredient:** Ashitaba adapts well to diverse culinary styles, whether fresh in salads, steeped in teas, or integrated into cooked recipes.

The use of Ashitaba in culinary techniques goes beyond its medical properties. Its versatility in a variety of dishes, as well as the nutritional advantages it provides, makes it a fascinating and important addition to the daily diet, both in traditional Japanese cuisine and in modern culinary inventions.

CHAPTER 5

Cultivation And Harvesting

Ashitaba, technically known as Angelica keiskei, is a Japanese perennial plant nicknamed "Tomorrow's Leaf" owing to its quick growth. Understanding the growing and harvesting procedures of this beneficial plant is critical to ensuring a sustainable supply.

Growing Conditions

Soil and Climate:

Temperate temperatures are ideal for Ashitaba, although it may adapt to a variety of environments. It does, however, require well-drained, slightly acidic soil rich in organic materials. The plant can survive both full sun and moderate shade, although, in hotter climates, it may need shelter from extreme heat.

Seeds, root cuttings, and stem cuttings are all ways of propagation. Seeds may take several weeks to germinate and are often planted in a nursery bed before being transplanted. Root and stem cuttings may also be used to propagate plants and grow quicker than seeds.

Maintenance and Care:

Regular watering without flooding and organic fertilizing on an as-needed basis may encourage healthy development. Mulching helps to retain moisture and inhibits weed development around plants. Pruning older leaves promotes new development and contributes to plant health.

Harvesting Guidelines

Timing:
Ashitaba leaves may be taken when they reach a suitable size, which is normally between 13 and 18 inches in height, while younger leaves can still be

harvested for culinary purposes. Harvesting regularly promotes continued development.

Harvesting Method:

To harvest the leaves, cut the stems at a small angle using sharp scissors or pruning shears, enabling the plant to regrow. To encourage additional development, pick gently without causing harm to the plant's primary core.

Sustainability Practices

Rotation of Crops:

Crop rotation, which involves moving ashitaba plants every year or every growing season, is important for maintaining soil fertility and preventing disease.

Organic Agriculture:
Organic farming practices promote healthier plants while maintaining the natural environment by

reducing the usage of synthetic pesticides and fertilizers.

Conservation Initiatives:

Sustainable harvesting procedures include avoiding overexploiting the wild plant population and promoting cultivation to fulfill ashitaba demand while protecting its natural environment.

The Value of Sustainable Practices:

As the demand for ashitaba grows because of its multiple health advantages, it is critical to implement sustainable production and harvesting procedures. Overharvesting or unethical farming may deplete wild populations and degrade the ecosystem.

Cultivating and harvesting ashitaba requires environmental sensitivity, providing a balance between human demands and the preservation of nature's resources. We may enjoy the advantages of ashitaba while also ensuring its survival for future generations if we follow sustainable practices.

CHAPTER 6

Processing And Production

Ashitaba, also known technically as Angelica keiskei, is a fascinating plant with a long history of traditional usage and a wide range of possible health advantages. In this chapter, we look at the processing and manufacture of Ashitaba, as well as the techniques used to harness its nutritional and therapeutic characteristics for a variety of purposes.

Extraction Methods

1. **Extraction of Leaves:**

• **Water Extraction:** One typical approach is to soak Ashitaba leaves in hot water to create an infusion. This method preserves water-soluble substances such as phytonutrients and vitamins.

• **Alcohol Extraction:** Some formulations extract both water-soluble and alcohol-soluble components using alcohol, extending the range of extracted elements.

2. Powder Manufacturing:

• **Drying Techniques:** To retain nutritional value, leaves may be air-dried or treated to low-temperature drying procedures after harvesting. After drying, the dried leaves are crushed into a fine powder.

• **Freeze-Drying:** This procedure is well-known for retaining optimum nutritional content by eliminating moisture at low temperatures. It is often recommended for preserving the delicate phytochemicals of the plant.

Manufacturing Processes

1. Production of Supplements:

• **Capsules and Tablets:** Ashitaba is often processed into supplement forms, encapsulated, or compressed into tablets for ease of use and consistent dosing.

- **Liquid Extracts:** Liquid extracts are created by condensing Ashitaba components into a liquid form that may be added to drinks or consumed straight.

2. Product Development in the Culinary Industry:

- **Ashitaba Tea:** This tasty and nutrient-rich tea is made from dried Ashitaba leaves. The leaves may be consumed whole or powdered.

- **Food Additives:** Ashitaba powder is used to enhance the taste and nutritional value of a variety of food items, including energy bars, smoothies, and snacks.

Commercial Products

1. Nutraceuticals:

- **Ashitaba Capsules:** These capsules often contain concentrated Ashitaba extract, making it easy to complement one's diet with its nutrients.

• **Multivitamin Formulas:** Ashitaba is sometimes used in multivitamin supplements, adding to the product's overall nutritional profile.

2. Culinary Options:

• **Ashitaba-Infused Products:** Some firms make culinary goods infused with Ashitaba, such as salad dressings, sauces, and spice mixes, which provide a distinctive and healthful touch to traditional dishes.

• **Ashitaba Tea Blends:** A variety of Ashitaba teas are available, some of which are mixed with other herbs or botanicals to appeal to a wide range of tastes.

CHAPTER 7

Health Benefits

Immune System Support

Ashitaba, also known as Angelica keiskei or "Tomorrow's Leaf," has gotten a lot of interest because of its possible immune-boosting effects. Ashitaba, which is rich in antioxidants, flavonoids, and vitamins, helps to strengthen the immune system greatly.

This plant's key components, including chalcones and xanthoangelol, have promising immunomodulatory properties, supporting the body in fighting infections and disorders. Regular ingestion may strengthen the body's natural defenses, lowering the probability of illness.

Digestive Health

Ashitaba has long been used to improve intestinal health. It includes chalcones and fibers, which help with digestion and intestinal health. These chemicals may aid in the regulation of digestive processes, the relief of gastrointestinal pain, and the improvement of nutritional absorption. Furthermore, the inclusion of prebiotic fibers promotes the development of good gut bacteria, leading to an overall better digestive system.

Anti-Inflammatory Properties

Ashitaba's anti-inflammatory properties are ascribed to its high phytonutrient content, which includes chalcones and flavonoids. These chemicals have anti-inflammatory characteristics that may aid in the treatment of inflammatory disorders such as arthritis, joint pain, and certain skin problems. Ashitaba may be able to lower inflammation by blocking inflammatory pathways, providing alleviation, and improving overall well-being.

Ashitaba has been shown in studies to have the capacity to modulate a variety of biological processes, including:

• **Antioxidant Activity:** Ashitaba contains antioxidants such as vitamins A, C, and E, which fight free radicals while also lowering oxidative stress and cellular damage.

• **Cardiovascular Support:** Ashitaba compounds have shown promise in improving heart health by possibly decreasing cholesterol levels and maintaining healthy circulation.

• **Blood Sugar Regulation:** Some studies show that Ashitaba may help regulate blood sugar levels, which might be beneficial for diabetics.

While these trials indicate promise, additional study is needed to demonstrate Ashitaba's entire spectrum of health benefits and effective doses for particular illnesses.

Integrating Ashitaba into one's diet, whether via teas, supplements, or culinary creations, may provide an easy approach to getting access to its possible health benefits. However, it is best to contact a healthcare expert before consuming Ashitaba for medicinal reasons, particularly if you have pre-existing medical issues or are taking drugs.

As more study is conducted, the potential health advantages of Ashitaba continue to pique the curiosity of traditional medicine practitioners as well as contemporary researchers, providing a promising route for holistic health and wellbeing.

CHAPTER 8

Potential Risks And Precautions

Allergies And Side Effects

1. **Allergic Reactions:** While uncommon, some people may be allergic to Ashitaba, especially if they are allergic to plants in the Apiaceae family, which includes carrots, parsley, and celery. Skin rashes, itching, and breathing problems are all possible symptoms.

2. **Gastrointestinal Distress:** Excessive use of Ashitaba or its supplements may cause minor gastrointestinal discomfort, such as diarrhea or nausea, in some people. Consumption should be done with caution.

Interactions With Medications

1. Blood-Thinning Medicines: Coumarins, which are found in Ashitaba, have modest blood-thinning characteristics. Individuals using anticoagulant drugs such as warfarin should take care while taking Ashitaba owing to the possibility of interactions that might increase the risk of bleeding.

2. Diabetes Medications: Ashitaba may reduce blood sugar levels. People on diabetic treatments, such as insulin or oral hypoglycemics, should closely check their blood sugar levels while taking Ashitaba to prevent hypoglycemia.

Dosage Recommendations

1. Dose recommendations: There are currently no established dose recommendations for Ashitaba supplements or intake. It is best to stick to the manufacturer's recommended dosages or consult with a healthcare professional for personalized advice.

2. Begin with modest dosages: For people who are new to Ashitaba, beginning with modest dosages might assist in measuring individual tolerance and minimize unwanted responses.

Precautionary Steps

1. Consult a Healthcare Professional: Before incorporating Ashitaba into your diet or using it as a supplement, especially if you have pre-existing health conditions or are taking medications, it's critical to get tailored guidance from a healthcare expert.

2. Pregnancy and Breastfeeding: There is little information available on the safety of Ashitaba during pregnancy and breastfeeding. Pregnant or breastfeeding women should avoid Ashitaba or consult a healthcare provider before using it.

3. Quality and Source: Ensure that Ashitaba products are of high quality and come from a reliable source. Buying from reputable sources can help to reduce the risk of contamination or adulteration.

4. Moderation is essential with any supplement or new addition to the diet. Excessive use of any herbal supplement can have negative consequences.

In conclusion, while Ashitaba may provide a variety of potential health benefits, it is critical to proceed with caution, especially if you have underlying health conditions or are taking medications. Before using it, consult a healthcare professional to help mitigate potential risks and ensure its safe integration into your wellness routine.

CHAPTER 9

Folklore And Cultural Significance

Ashitaba, scientifically known as Angelica keiskei, is not only a valuable herb in terms of nutrition and health benefits, but it also has folklore and cultural significance. This chapter delves into Ashitaba's mythological references, cultural practices, and symbolic significance.

Mythological References

In many Asian cultures, Ashitaba is associated with mythology and folklore, and is often revered for its mystical properties. According to some myths, Ashitaba is a symbol of longevity and vitality. The plant's regenerative abilities, as well as its rapid growth and resilience, contribute to its depiction as a magical herb in myths and legends.

In Japanese folklore, Ashitaba is known as "Tomorrow's Leaf" or "Longevity Herb," implying a belief in its ability to promote a long and healthy life. The name Ashitaba translates to "Tomorrow's Leaf" in Japanese, emphasizing the idea that its consumption may lead to a healthier tomorrow.

Cultural Practices And Beliefs

Ashitaba has been used in traditional medicine and culinary practices throughout Asia. For centuries, it has been a part of traditional Japanese healing practices, believed to have the power to rejuvenate the body and promote overall well-being.

Ashitaba is associated with purification rituals in some cultures. Its use in ceremonial teas and infusions emphasizes its cultural significance as a symbol of cleansing and renewal.

Symbolic Importance

Ashitaba is more than just a plant; it has cultural significance. Because of its vibrant green leaves and distinct appearance, it has become a symbol of health, resilience, and hope. In some cultures, the plant is revered, and its cultivation and use are linked to spiritual beliefs.

Ashitaba's symbolism encompasses broader themes of renewal and regeneration. Its ability to grow quickly and thrive in a variety of environments has led to its association with the life, death, and rebirth cycle. Because of this symbolic resonance, Ashitaba has been included in a variety of cultural ceremonies and rituals.

Understanding Ashitaba's folklore and cultural significance expands its identity beyond its nutritional and medicinal properties. The intertwining of mythology, cultural practices, and symbolic meanings reflects the rich tapestry of human interactions with the natural world, in which plants like Ashitaba serve as carriers of cultural heritage and beliefs as well as resources.

CHAPTER 10

Future Research And Developments

Ashitaba, scientifically known as Angelica keiskei, is a revered plant in traditional Japanese medicine and cuisine, celebrated for its numerous benefits and adaptability. Several intriguing avenues for exploring and expanding our understanding of this remarkable plant exist in the realm of future research and development.

Ongoing Studies

1. **Biomedical Research:** Current research focuses on the biologically active compounds found in Ashitaba. Researchers want to find and isolate specific phytochemicals that are responsible for the plant's medicinal properties, such as chalcones, flavonoids, and coumarins. Understanding these

compounds at the molecular level can provide information about their therapeutic potential.

2. Clinical Trials: Continuous clinical trials seek to validate traditional claims while also discovering new therapeutic applications. Ashitaba's effects on various health aspects, such as immune modulation, anti-inflammatory properties, digestive health, and potential uses in managing chronic conditions like diabetes or cardiovascular disease, are being investigated.

3. Nutritional Studies: The nutritional composition of Ashitaba is of interest. Ongoing research aims to map out its vitamins, minerals, amino acids, and antioxidants to understand how these constituents contribute to its health benefits.

Potential Discoveries

1. **Bioactive Compounds:** Further research into Ashitaba may reveal novel bioactive compounds with unique medicinal properties. The discovery of these compounds could lead to the creation of new pharmaceuticals or nutraceuticals.

2. **Synergistic Effects:** Researching Ashitaba in conjunction with other herbs or medicines may reveal synergistic effects, potentially increasing its efficacy in treating a variety of health conditions. Understanding these interactions has the potential to transform treatment protocols.

3. **Genetic Research:** Researching the plant's genetics may lead to the cultivation of more potent or disease-resistant varieties. This could improve cultivation practices while also increasing the quality and quantity of bioactive compounds found in Ashitaba.

Areas For Further Exploration

1. **Long-Term Effects:** Long-term research into the effects of Ashitaba consumption is critical. Understanding its long-term impact can provide insights into its safety and efficacy for long-term use.

2. **Standardization and Quality Control:** By establishing standardized extraction methods and quality control measures, Ashitaba-based products are more consistent. This includes determining the best harvesting times, processing techniques, and storage conditions for the bioactive compounds.

3. Beyond its known health benefits, researching Ashitaba's potential applications in skin care, veterinary medicine, or as a functional food ingredient could open new markets and expand its usage.

4. **Cultivation Methods:** It is critical to develop sustainable and efficient cultivation methods to

meet rising demand while maintaining the plant's ecological integrity. This includes investigating optimal growing conditions, organic farming practices, and environmentally friendly harvesting methods.

The future of Ashitaba research is bright, not only in terms of revealing its untapped therapeutic potential but also in deepening our understanding of its cultural significance and ecological role. As science continues to unravel its mysteries, Ashitaba is poised to make even greater contributions to human health and well-being while honoring its rich cultural heritage.

Conclusion

We've delved into Ashitaba's multifaceted aspects in this comprehensive journey, uncovering a tapestry woven with tradition, science, and cultural significance. Ashitaba, also known as "Tomorrow's Leaf," embodies a trove of virtues, displaying a range of nutritional, medicinal, and cultural profundities that transcend time and borders.

Summary Of Key Points

The nutritional profile of Ashitaba emerged as a cornerstone throughout our investigation. It is high in vitamins and minerals such as vitamins A, B, C, and calcium, as well as phytonutrients, which explains its potent antioxidant properties. This combination makes it a force to be reckoned with when it comes to boosting immunity, improving digestive health, and combating inflammation.

Ashitaba's medicinal uses shed light on its evolution from traditional healing practices to modern medicinal applications. From its historical reverence as a natural remedy to its incorporation into modern medicine, scientific studies and ongoing research have substantiated its efficacy in health-related domains.

Culinary traditions have incorporated Ashitaba seamlessly, infusing its essence into a variety of recipes and culinary tips. Its versatility in dishes, beverages, and supplements provides not only a gustatory delight but also a nutritional boon, allowing for easy incorporation into daily diets.

The complexities of Ashitaba cultivation and harvesting highlight its sustainable growth practices, thriving under specific environmental conditions while adhering to ethical harvesting guidelines. This balanced approach ensures its continued availability while also preserving its natural habitat.

THE END